Cosmic Readings
for
Hatha Yoga

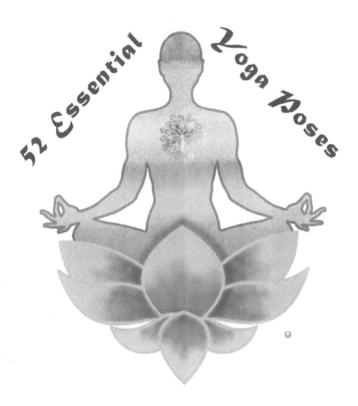

52 Essential Yoga Poses

Gianna Ragona-Suarez

ISBN: 9781791622183

Dear Reader;
I send you blessings and deep gratitude for
holding this book in your hands. This book is a
compilation of readings, some of my own and
those inspired and written by others. They are my
favorites and I wish you the same success reading
them during and after your yoga practice. My
students have loved them and asked for copies,
hence the creation of this book.
On the following pages you will find the basic and
essential poses of yoga. If you take your time in
each pose and read the meditation attributed to
the pose it will bring you gently into the MindBody
connection which is indeed the path of yoga.
To add to the MindBody connection always
remember to keep the breath long and deep
(emanating from the diaphragm and the ribcage)
this will bring your practice full circle into the
deepest expression of yoga

Namaste,
Gianna Ragona-Suarez

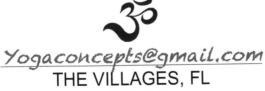

Yogaconcepts@gmail.com
THE VILLAGES, FL
11/27/2018

Cosmic Readings
for
Hatha Yoga

Compiled & Artwork
by
Gianna Ragona-Suarez

500hour E-RYT Experienced-Registered Yoga
Instructor and Yoga Teacher Trainer.

Poses

Readings

..... and finally...

Seated Easy Pose

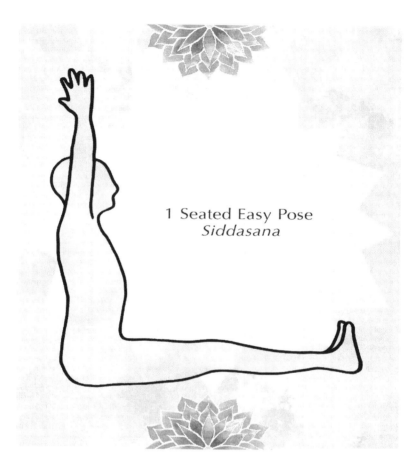

1 Seated Easy Pose
Siddasana

Calms the mind, prepares the body for an aligned
practice. Breath calmly, gaze ahead, arms aligned
alongside the ears.

Let Go Of Performing And Come Into Being

In yoga we let go of outward comparisons
Instead we practice inward focus and non-
competing,
We seek inner connection and integrate
States of movement into meditative oneness.
We slide into the domain of the spirit as
We breathe and move through our poses.
It is here where transformation and oneness
happen.
The unity of Yoga exudes beauty,
Then all becomes grace and flow.
We move as though inspired by water
But fueled by the sun.
We sit grounded on this earth we call home.
We gaze upward at endless sky and the divine.
We focus inward in our yoga practice
Unaware of all the souls who have come to share
this class.
We slide into the oneness of being without effort.
We let go of judgement, let go of comparison and
competition.
We hear and feel only the sound of our own
breath.
Gianna

Seated Lateral Stretch

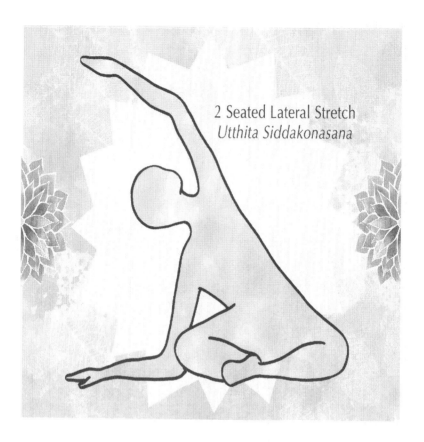

2 Seated Lateral Stretch
Utthita Siddakonasana

Stretches and elongates the side body. Rest hand or forearm on the earth as you gaze and reach the opposite arm skyward and over the ear.

The Science Of Yoga

Dr. Martin Rossman, MD UCSF

Yoga is hands down one of the best self-care tools.
Spending time on your mat can benefit your brain, heart and bones and even change the expression of your genetic makeup.
Science is uncovering new ways this ancient practice creates healthier lives.
We squeeze and cleanse our internal organs.
We lubricate our joints.
We move our bio chemistry around.
We breathe deeply exhaling toxins
And in the end, we spend quiet moments.
Allowing our bodies to metabolize all the new energy.
As we leave our mats and move out into the world
We are renewed and refreshed.

Seated Spinal Twist

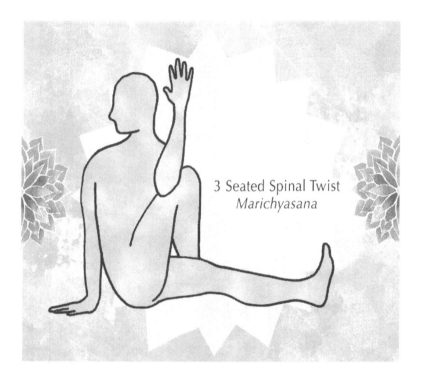

3 Seated Spinal Twist
Marichyasana

Keep the spine straight and elongated, Bring the elbow to push against the outside of the knee. Gaze over the back shoulder.

Peace Be With You

May today, there be peace within.
May you **trust** that you are exactly where you are
meant to be.
May you not forget the infinite possibilities that are
born of faith in yourself and in others.
May you use the gifts that you have received and
pass on the love that has been given you.
May you be content with yourself just the way you
are.
Let this knowledge settle into your bones and
allow your soul the freedom
to sing, dance, praise and love!
It is there for each and every one of us.
May the peace of the universe guide and bless
you.
May you share this peace and blessings with
others.
Unknown Author

Cat/Cow Spinal Stretch

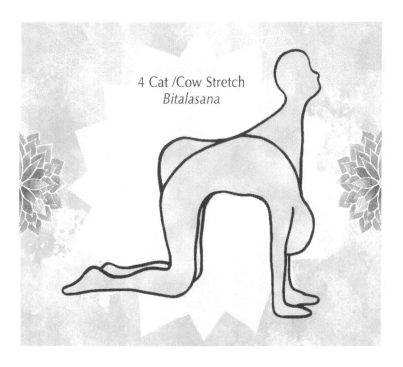

4 Cat /Cow Stretch
Bitalasana

Awakens and lubricates the spine. Classic warm-up for beginning the practice.

This Is What I Have To Say To You
By Danna Faulds

This is what I have to say to you . . .
Live as if the earth exhales blessings in your
direction,
As if trees speak their deepest secrets In your ear,
As if bird songs can lift you outside your
Ordinary state of mind and bring you into truth.
Be the creative juice flowing through the universe.
Be compassion in action and wholeness in motion.
Be silence and stillness, the ocean of love so
Palpable that not one cell of you disputes
the truth that you are love.
Be so open to your destiny that it
Unfurls like a banner in the sky, saying,
"Live with gratitude, generosity, and grace."

Sunbird Pose

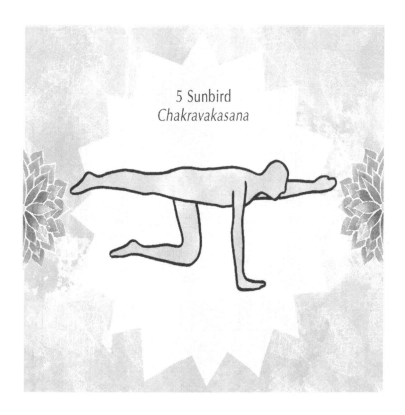

5 Sunbird
Chakravakasana

Creates balance, builds core, glutes and shoulder strength. Gaze is steady ahead, breath is long and even.

Within This Body You Are Wearing
By Robert Hall

Within this body you are wearing,
Now inside the bones and beating in the heart,
Lives the one you have been searching for so
long.
But you must stop running away and shake hands.
The meeting doesn't happen
Without your presence . . . your participation.
The same one waiting for you there
Is moving in the trees, glistening on the water,
Growing in the grasses
And lurking in the shadows you create.
You have nowhere to go.
The marriage happened long ago.
Behold your mate lives within you.

Mountain Pose

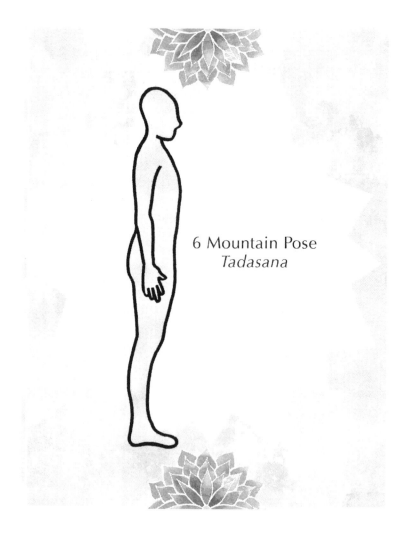

6 Mountain Pose
Tadasana

Strong, rooted, spine aligned, tailbone reaching earthward. Strength in being grounded.

The Seekers

You who are the seeker…
Whatever path you are on
has brought you here to this moment….

Soon the Divine pulsation grabs you
And carries you into its dance.
In the midst of ecstatic motion,
Your body dissolves into light leaving only the
softly glowing benediction of the bones.

You become serene within, eyes open in
amazement,
Seeing the unseen vastness into the nectar of
eternity
The soul reveals itself to itself.

Through breath infused movement, twists,
stretches, balances, the hand, foot, spine…
Your form aligns with mind, heart and voice.

The invisible become visible to eyes that look
within.
Now you discover that YOU are the one you have
been seeking.

Standing Crescent Pose

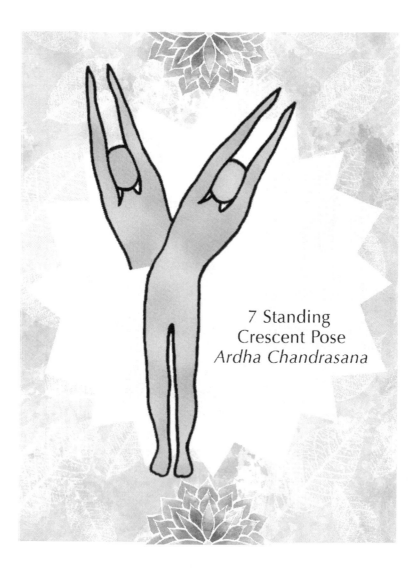

7 Standing
Crescent Pose
Ardha Chandrasana

Arms alongside the ears, spine is straight, hips push to one side as the arms reach in opposite direction, glutes, core engaged.

You Are Part Of All

Sit in any relaxed, comfortable pose.
Experience the support of the earth below
As substantial but ever changing,
As minute particles in ecstatic motion.

Feel support below, feel support from above
Feel support for the movement of hands and feet,
Feel support for the mind.
Be completely at peace knowing you are part of all
That exists on this planet.

Remembering that you are a child of the universe.
Gianna

Forward Fold

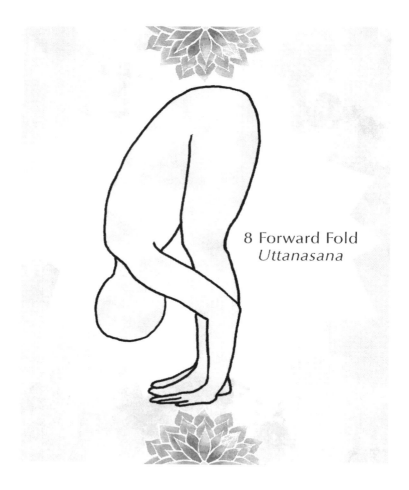

8 Forward Fold
Uttanasana

Hinging at the hips, be patient with yourself as you
spine lengthens toward the earth. Heaviness of
the head elongates and unclenches the spine.
Soften your knees if necessary until the
hamstrings find release.

The Embrace

Oceans embrace a continent,
Space welcomes the sun,
Earth holds you to her bosom with its gravity.

Lose yourself in this generosity.

Form your arms into a circle,
Bow to the energy of the sun,
Rise to flat back to absorb energy into the spine.

Cherish the arising of serenity and devotion.
Attend the birth of something new.
Celebrate the seedling's spring arrival.

Let thoughts dissolve into peace.
The ripples of the lake come to stillness
The wind in the trees remain unbroken and
constant,
As you become the one who embraces all of life.
Danna Faulds

Chair Pose

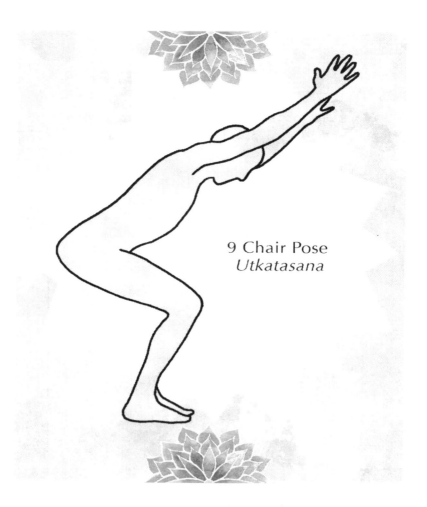

9 Chair Pose
Utkatasana

Works the back, thighs, shoulders and mind as you persevere into this pose.

Go In And In
Danna Faulds

Go in and in.
Be the space between two cells,
The vast, resounding silence in which
Spirit dwells.
Be sugar dissolving on the tongue of life.

Dive in and in,
As deep as you can dive.
Be infinite, ecstatic truth.

Be love conceived and born in union.
Be exactly what you seek,
Be the Beloved, singing "Yes",
Tasting "Yes", embracing "Yes",

Until there is only essence of the all
Of everything expressing through you
As you go in and in.

High Crescent Lunge

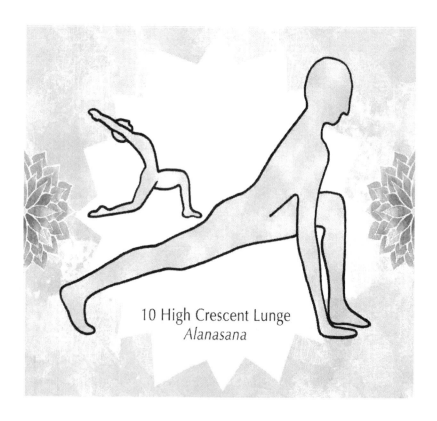

10 High Crescent Lunge
Alanasana

Back leg strong, muscles engaged, stay on the ball of the back foot, when you feel secure raise and extend your arms skyward. Fix your gaze to keep your balance.

The Inner Teacher - Sva Guru

The Inner Teacher is the best teacher you will ever
have!
In Sanskrit known as the Sva Guru!
Much of yoga practice is about
learning to honor and
listen to one's inner teacher.
After all, the very practice of yoga is an
Inward journey.
The outer healer has a role too, the doctor, the
therapist, the surgeon,
But the most important healer is the one inside.

The role of a good yoga teacher is to guide
and support students with knowledge,
skill and loving compassion
into self-knowing
and into trusting their inner teacher.

You the student, then become the **Sva Guru.**
Your own Inner Teacher

Om to the Inner Teacher….
Together we chant….
Om Sva Guru, Om Sva Guru, Om Sva Guru
Gianna

Five Pointed Star

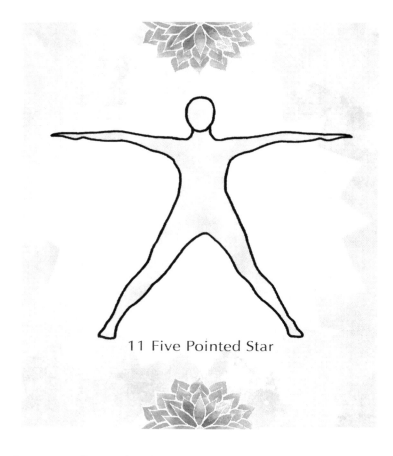

11 Five Pointed Star

A pose of gentle determination, keep your limbs
extended, gaze fixed, arms shoulder height. Hold
and breath, feel where your body is in space.
Proprioception.

Life Changes, We Are Resilient

The yogic thinking is that there's part of us that's
unchanging. Deep inside of us the spiritual side has
infinite peace and joy and love.
The nature of the world, however, is in flux.
Learning to make peace with life's calamities —
lost jobs, broken marriage, lost dreams—
does not mean you have to be passive.
You can soothe the discomfort brought on by external
changes through having faith in the process that
brings equanimity and peace, our yoga practice shows
us how.
We practice mindfulness so that we can be guided
from within. In stilling our thoughts, we free up a more
reliable inner wisdom. The more peaceful the mind is,
the clearer and stronger our intuition is, and the better
able we are to make the proper decision. We create a
deeper reserve to call upon when life changes
direction. When we learn to go with the universal flow
and allow the good intention to lead us we find clarity
and meaning. Maybe you were meant to lose that job
so you can move onto another, better job. Maybe the
divorce means ending a toxic situation and finding
peace deep within. Maybe the kids moving away will
give you more free time to write that book.
Instead of dwelling on what has been lost, look for the
**new you out there. Embody and embrace the
opportunity that has been given you.**

Warrior 1

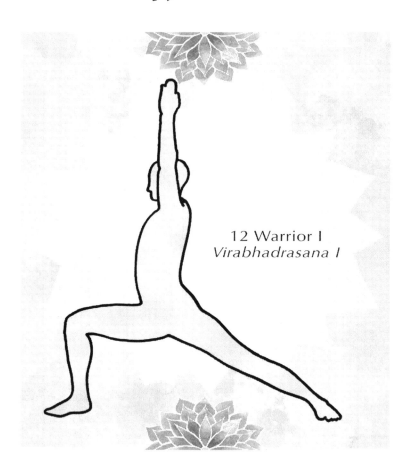

12 Warrior I
Virabhadrasana I

The Warrior Virabhadra was revered for his steady strength and fierceness. Back foot firmly rooted, front thigh parallel to the earth, gaze fixed, breath deep and steady.

Space Within And Without

Gaze out at space
See the multicolored luminosity which permeates
everywhere.
The blue sky filled with rays from the sun.
The bright white of the clouds.
Find wonder in how infinite it is.

Come home to your true self,
Expansive, bright, multicolored, permeating
everywhere, radiating within and without.

Gaze at the night sky, dark yet crisscrossed by the
light of a billion stars
How can it be that all space is the same,
Inside of you and far away?
Lose yourself in this spaciousness.
Danna Faulds

Reverse Warrior

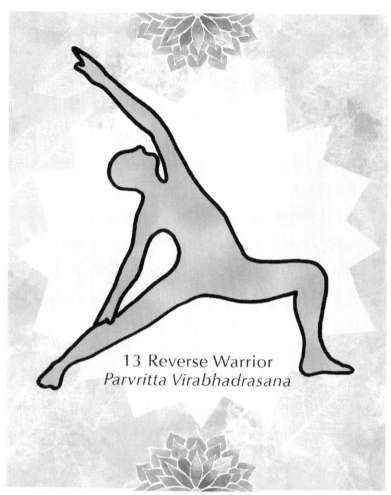

13 Reverse Warrior
Parvritta Virabhadrasana

As Warrior reaches behind to recoil the ribcage is stretched, arm elongated, legs firm, muscles engaged, he prepares for battle.

Surfing Life's Turbulent Waters

We can't stop the waves from coming in and out of
our lives, but we can learn to skillfully surf them
when they roll our way.
Not surprisingly, these are skills one learns
through meditation and yoga breath.
We begin by learning to trust life.

Nature teaches us that there are cycles to life:
beginnings, middles, evolutions and endings.
Knowing this helps us to feel more at rest with the
knowledge that things will, in fact, **change**.
If you breathe deeply and have patience,
all things pass.
Remember, you are a Child of the Universe and
the Universe is here to guide and help you.

The personal faith in yourself has much to do with
your success during these turbulent times.
With your breath and confidence you can weather
any storm.

Warrior 2

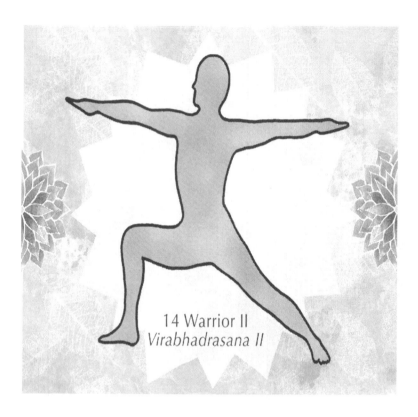

14 Warrior II
Virabhadrasana II

Warrior II, stretches horizontally, legs engaged,
gaze fixed on the target, quiet determination.

In The Stillness Between Breath – Kumbaka

We clear out the clutter, downsize the
possessions.
Find room for silent time.
It is then that we find that stillness between
breaths.
In that space when the body is
Between inhale and exhale…
This stillness called "Kumbaka".

Kumbaka gives us great insight, it calms the
parasympathetic system,
Bringing the body to momentary stillness.
So, rest in Kumbaka, that is where the secrets lie.

You are hereby authorized to let go
of that stuff that has weighed you down.
You are hereby authorized to become all you care
to be.
Kumbaka gives us the vision needed to see the
pure light of ourselves in that moment of stillness.
Gianna

Extended Side Angle Warrior

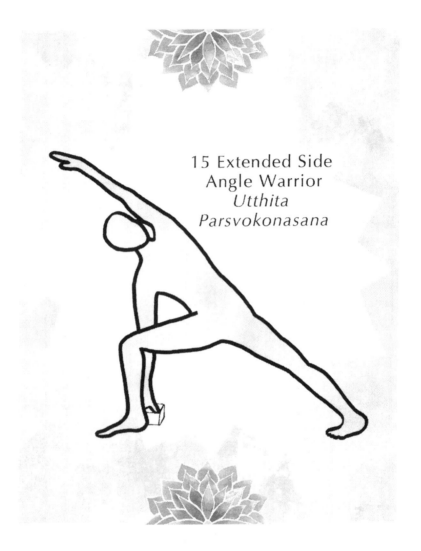

15 Extended Side
Angle Warrior
*Utthita
Parsvokonasana*

Find balance in stretching laterally, create the
strong powerful straight line of energy from ankle
to wrist. Breath fully.

Just For Now
Dana Faulds

Just for now, without asking how,
Let yourself sink into stillness.
Just for now, lay down the
weight you so patiently
bear upon your shoulders.

Feel the earth receive you,
and allow the infinite expanse of sky
grow even wider as your awareness
reaches up to meet it.

Just for now, allow a wave of breath
to enliven your experience.
Breathe out whatever blocks you
From the truth.

Just for now, be boundless, free,
Awakened energy tingling in your
hands and feet.

Drink in the possibility of being
who and what you really are!
Be so fully alive that when you
open your eyes the world looks
different, newly born and vibrant,
just for now.

Triangle Pose

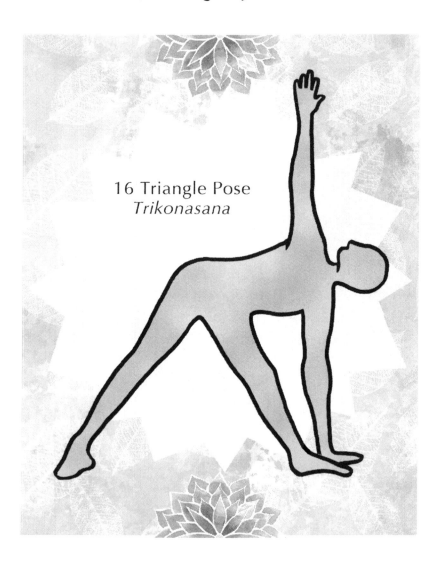

16 Triangle Pose
Trikonasana

Arms form one straight powerful line, legs are
straight, firmly rooted, gaze is skyward.

The Cherokee Tale Of 2 Wolves

There is an ancient tale the Chief once told his grandson about a fight going on inside of him.

He said to the boy "There is a terrible fight within me between two wolves. One is evil, he is anger, envy, sorry, regret, greed, arrogance, self-pity, resentment, inferiority, lies, false pride, superiority, self-doubt and ego.
The other is good, he is joy, peace, love, hope, serenity, humility, kindness, benevolence, empathy, generosity, truth, compassion and faith. "

He said, "The same fight is going on inside of you, and inside of every other person too."

The grandson thought about it for a minute and then asked his grandfather, "Which will win?"

The old Chief simply replied, "The one who wins is the one you feed."

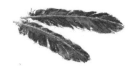

Downward Facing Dog

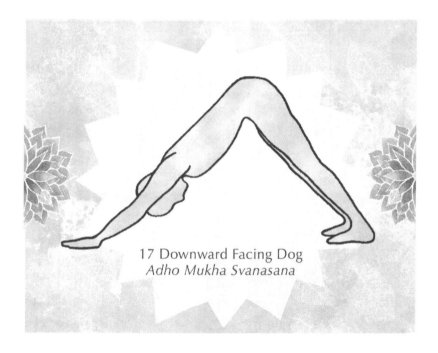

17 Downward Facing Dog
Adho Mukha Svanasana

The quintessential pose, encompasses so many benefits. Upper body strength, hamstrings stretch, inversion sends energy to the brain, heart takes a rest as it is lower than the other organs, back elongates, spine releases, shoulders tone. Deep breathing seals the pose.

Finding Balance Through Yoga

The only ingredients we can rely on to experience balance is our own body, speech, breath and mind.

We'd like to think we can rely on external situations, the house, a job, our children…as if they were unchanging.
But none of these elements are fixed entities and when we grasp at them for security, we lose the opportunity for a balanced life.
The kids will grow up and leave, you may get downsized at work, and your plumbing – both in your house and in your body can spring a leak without warning. Nothing is solid. Even the planet we live on is hurling through space.

Rather than going through life on auto-pilot, counting on everything staying the same and then getting hit with surprises, by familiarizing ourselves with the rhythms of our own body, breath and mind, we can learn how to sail through our life no matter what the weather report.
Cyndy Lee, founder of Om Studio

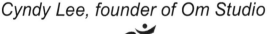

Warrior 3 Balance

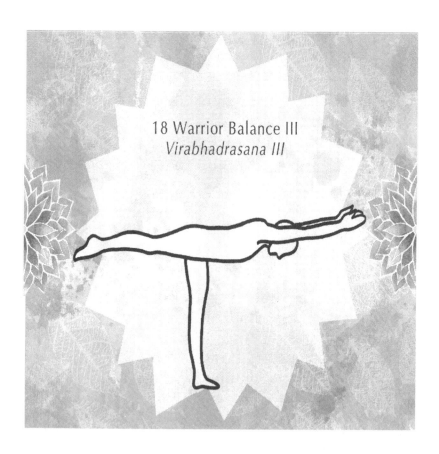

18 Warrior Balance III
Virabhadrasana III

Challenge your ability to balance, strongly engage the standing leg, reach arms alongside ears, lengthen and breathe. Find your dristhti on the floor.

Pranayama Offers Great Expansion Of Your Life Force

Its gifts come when you become "one" with the flow of the breath and movement.
Organically, your body senses the calmness of the inhalation and exhalation used in yoga practice.
Ujjayi is a deep resonate breath emanating from the diaphragm, up the ribcage, through the chest, the back of the throat almost as a snore.
This breath brings us to full presence and the sound of it pulls us into harmony with those around us.

Pay attention the next time you are sitting with a friend or loved one, pay attention and you will notice that **if you are connected** you will likely be breathing together.

As a teacher, listening to a room full of yogis, I have felt what it is like to have my breath connected to each and every person in the room.
We are all organically breathing audibly, in unison and it becomes a beautiful flow of energy and power.
It is called Ujjayi Breath, it informs and powers up our practice.
Gianna

Wide Stance Forward Fold

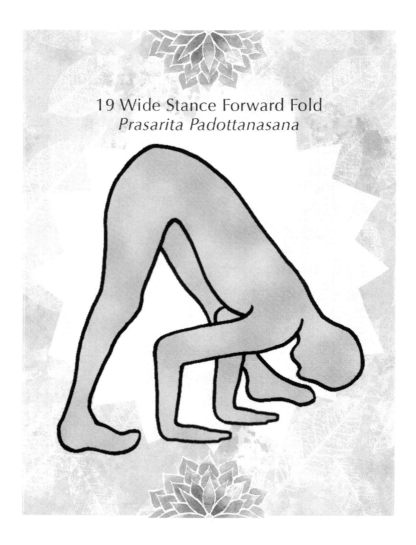

19 Wide Stance Forward Fold
Prasarita Padottanasana

This inversion stretches hamstrings, sends a rush of energy to the brain, moves the biochemistry around in the body, changes your perspective of the room around you.

In Forward Fold

Hinging from the hips and diving into forward fold,
we move the bio-chemistry around in our bodies.
We allow a rush of fresh energy to ignite the brain
and therefore the consciousness.
If we open our eyes in forward fold and look
around the room we see things in a new
perspective, our world appears upside down but
perfectly normal.
Our brain registers the moment and the view as
something perfectly acceptable.

In the end, we realize that this flexibility of view
makes us calm and brings us to an acceptance of
things as they are in the outside world even if they
are for the moment, upside down.

Our perspective of the world has changed and
therefore our ability to accept, adapt and view
things differently. We refresh our thinking and
broaden our understanding.
Gianna

Forward Fold Twist

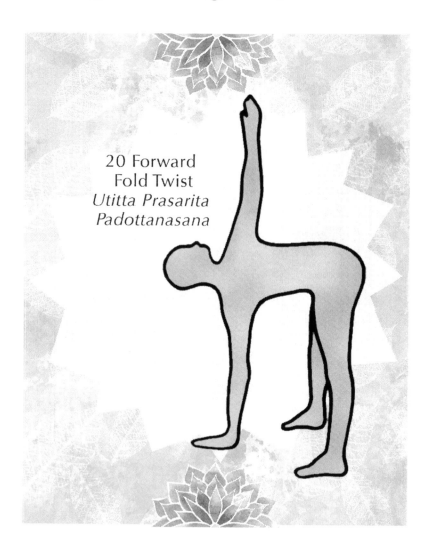

20 Forward
Fold Twist
*Utitta Prasarita
Padottanasana*

Place one hand under your face, draw the
opposite hand skyward as you twist and turn your
gaze toward your upper hand. Legs are wide
apart, feet rooted. Lubricates spine.

Why Do You Stand There In All Your Doubt?
Peg Mulqueen

Why do you stand there in all your doubt?
Don't you know that your whole life has led you to
this moment...preparing you?
Your feet have grown rooted and firm...
The result of all those storms you weathered.
Yours are the feet that stand their ground.
Your legs are powerful...
A strength built from trudging through some rough
and dangerous terrain. Yours are the legs that
move mountains.
Your shoulders are broad... as they are practiced
in carrying not only the load you have been given
but often bearing the bundle of another.
Yours are the shoulders that hold others up.
All the tears you shed have cleared your vision...
Giving you a greater capacity to see all that is
there... and who are there before you.
Yours are the eyes that not only look into the eyes
of another but into the heart of another as well. ...
And your heart, my friend, has only grown
bigger... each time it was broken and patched
back together. Yours is the heart that no longer
knows limits in its capacity to love.
Even your hands are not the hands you began
with... For now their grasp is tighter and grip is
stronger. Yours are the hands of understanding.
I know you are shaking, its true.....

The challenge that lies before is like none you've
faced before.
I know you are tired, and you should be.
You've struggled long and hard to get where you
stand now.
But I promise you, that all you've endured or
enjoyed, relished in or suffered with, each time
you won....but even more the times you didn't,
have all played their part in escorting you to this
place....
Your edge.
And it is not the place you stop....
Oh No, my friend, it's the place from which you'll
begin.

Rise Above & Overcome Self Doubt

Whenever you find yourself doubting how far you can go in life,
Remember how far you have already come.
The trials you've had to face.
The trials and tribulations you've already been through.
The battles you've had to fight
And the fears you've had to overcome.
The road not taken was not taken for a reason.
Have faith in your ability to overcome.
Trust that you are exactly where you are meant to be.
Trust that you are exactly where you are meant to be.

Childs Pose

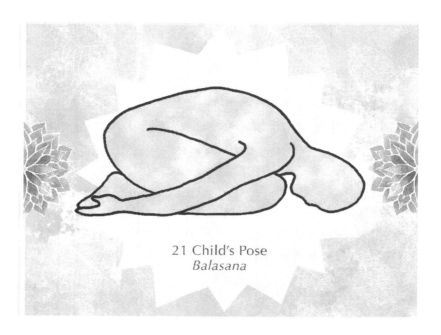

21 Child's Pose
Balasana

Ultimate resting pose. Feel the stretch along the
spine, rest forehead on the earth, hands palms up,
breathing quiet and calm.

The Body-Mind Connection

In yogic terms, there is no separation between mind, body and spirit.
The three exist as one, a "union" (definition of the word *yoga*).
What happens to the mind also happens to the body and spirit and so on. In other words, if something is bothering you spiritually, emotionally, or mentally, it is likely to show up in your body.
And as you work deeply with your body in yoga, emotional issues will likely come to the fore.
In the yogic view, we all hold within our bodies emotions and misguided thoughts that keep us from reaching *samadhi*, "conscious enlightenment".
Any sense of unease or dis-ease in the body keeps us from reaching and experiencing this state of enlightenment.
Asanas (poses) are a path to blissful contentment, working to bring us closer by focusing our minds and releasing any emotional or inner tension in our bodies.
This practice brings us to the knowledge that there is no separation between mind, body and spirit but rather we are the sum total of Mind/Body/Spirit & Breath.
Gianna

Cobra Pose

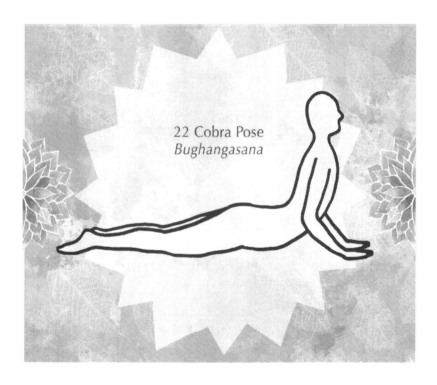

22 Cobra Pose
Bughangasana

In cobra, arms remain bent, belly resting on the earth as the chest pushes forward. Shoulders drop away from the ears. Spine is relaxed, gaze is steady.

Yoga Practice Is A Workshop For Our Lives!

We learn to breathe through various odd shapes and poses, we maintain our balance and equilibrium, we practice non-harming, we show compassion to ourselves and others.
What better training ground is there than our yoga practice?

In the age of corporate everything, profit becomes more important than product, and so it seems to be with yoga.

But yoga is a complete system, and when practiced sincerely and regularly over a long period of time the result is an improved quality of life.

If the practice of pranayama and yogic philosophy are removed it can lead to a state of imbalance rather than peace. Brought together all of these qualities of yoga practice create an effortless rhythm to life. The space and time on our mats gives us the training required to move off the mat and out into the world with renewed vision and energy.
Gianna

Plank Pose

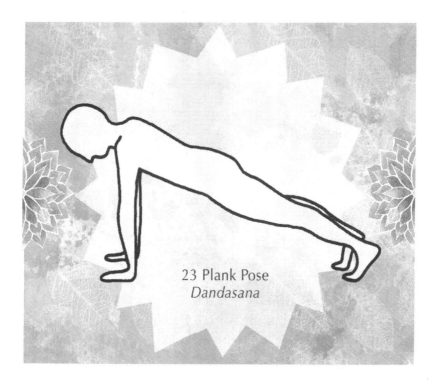

23 Plank Pose
Dandasana

Building upper body and core strength, hold firm
and straight from the back of the head to the
heels. Keep the spine long, do not let the head fall
toward the earth but keep the neck long. Broaden
shoulders, breathe deeply. Hold for 10 breaths.

In Yoga We Work On The Interior As Well As The Exterior

By building inner and outer strength, shifting from
fearful to courageous, we discover that Yoga helps
us navigate change and transformation.
Simply by understanding that all things change,
winter becomes spring, becomes summer,
becomes fall, then becomes winter again.
Our brown hair becomes grey, our children grow
and leave the nest.
Change is the constant dynamic power of life.
When we are stagnant or stuck, we find ourselves
in an attitude of resistance, which leaves us
stunted from growth.
The various physical states of your life flow as the
seasons and the tides in a dance of up and down
along with the flow of thoughts and emotions.
We navigate with ease when we learn to breathe,
surrender, meditate and honor the changes and
ride through with equanimity and grace.
Baron Baptiste

Low Lunge, Knee to Floor

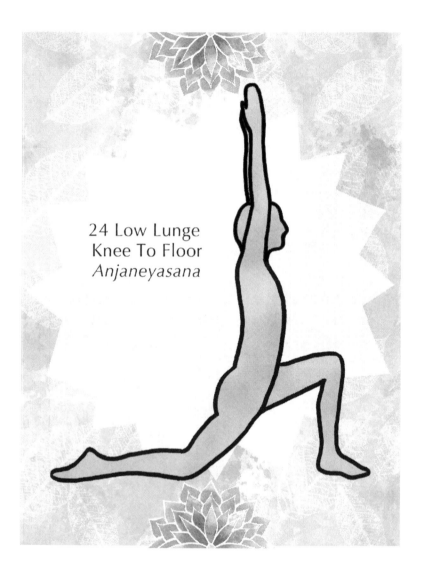

24 Low Lunge
Knee To Floor
Anjaneyasana

The back knee rests on the earth while the torso
and arms reach skyward. Keep the spine straight.
Breath into the length.

Springtime - Clearing Away The Rocks

The springtime is the season of *TRANSFORMATION*; we are released from the lethargy of winter. We begin with removing the rocks from our garden, the rocks that blocked our progress and kept us from realizing our true potential.
By removing the rocks of anger, pride, fear, resistance, we come back to our natural way of being, which is free, happy, almost innocent in our vision of the world.
If you are free of judgment then all things will appear fresh and new, you will embrace more and learn more.
We can begin to blossom to the diverse dynamics around us. Our ground will be fertile for planting of new ideas, service to others, fresh goals and abundance.
Transformation comes not by adding things but by removing debris and negative thoughts that didn't belong there in the first place.
We change by peeling away layers of old, outworn habits and beliefs. The old habit of looking outside of ourselves for things that will prove our worth will not fix or satisfy us.
Within us lies all that we really need and it nourishes and shines through when the rocks of the garden are cleared away.

Pyramid Pose

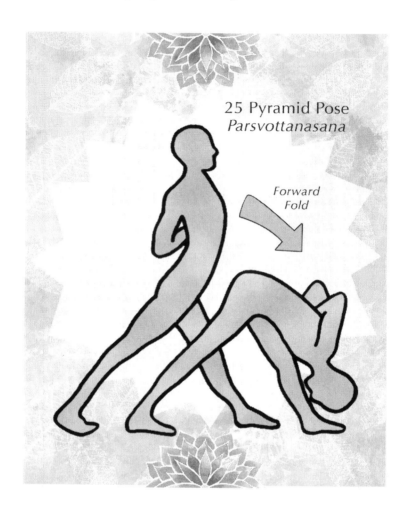

25 Pyramid Pose
Parsvottanasana

Forward
Fold

Sweep your arms behind you and clasp the elbow
or interlace your fingers. Lift chest skyward then
hinge at the forward hip as you lengthen the spine
hinging forward into a forward fold. See how close
you can get you nose to your knee. Then peel
back up.

Alignment In Your Poses

If your car is out of alignment, you can still drive it,
but eventually the tires wear unevenly putting
stress on other parts of the vehicle. It becomes an
accident waiting to happen.
By the same token, if you enter your poses out of
alignment you do not receive the benefit of the
pose but more importantly you stress other areas
of your body.
If the hips are not stable under the shoulders and
the front knee is not aligned over the front ankle
then the Warrior poses becomes a wasted effort,
nothing is gained.
Make your efforts count by adjusting into
alignment. Your body will tell you what and how.
Gianna

Half Moon Balance

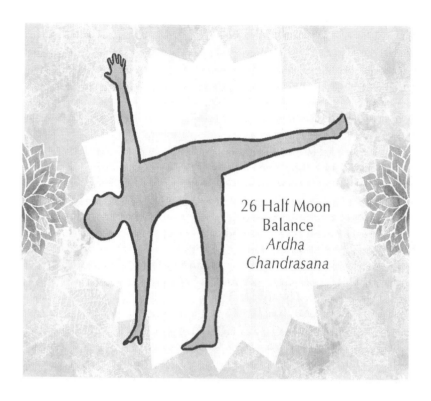

26 Half Moon
Balance
*Ardha
Chandrasana*

From 3 point balance, find your drishti, strengthen
the standing leg then begin to slowly raise the
opposite leg and arm skyward. Breathe, keep the
gaze firm.

Practice Steady Effort "Abhyasa"

So, when you are starting on your life change, consider the steps you need to take to make it happen through the technique of "Self-Inquiry". Creating these small, stepping stones of action a little at a time will help you to avoid feeling overwhelmed.

Consider the slow steady progress of the turtle, remember, that he never makes progress until he sticks his neck out.

In this process of shedding and "letting go" is important. If you keep going back and reassessing the old situation you will expend your energy needlessly.

When instead, you "let go", your mind and creative energies are free to experience what is new and available to you.

As you breathe out allow the letting go to release out all that no longer serves you.

As you do this, you will experience a freedom that comes with growth.

These are the inner keys to radical change.

You will find yourself receiving the greatest gift of change, rebirth, coming closer to the life of your dreams, free of anxiety, full of light, energy and curiosity.

Welcome to the next chapter, your soul awaits you.

Gate Pose

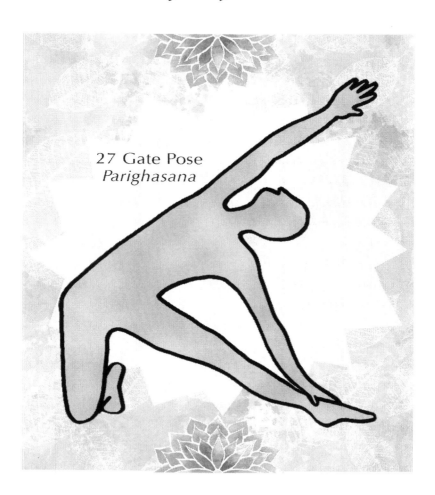

27 Gate Pose
Parighasana

From kneeling, extend one leg away, root that foot into the mat. Begin to hinge sideways over the extended leg, place hand on the foot or ankle (never on the knee). Reach skyward with the upper arm, gaze skyward, breathe.

Mother Teresa's *Anyway* Poem

People are often unreasonable, illogical and self-centered;
Forgive them anyway.
If you are kind, people may accuse you of selfish, ulterior motives;
Be kind anyway.
If you are successful, you will win some false friends and some true enemies;
Succeed anyway.
If you are honest and frank, people may cheat you;
Be honest and frank anyway.
What you spend years building, someone could destroy overnight;
Build anyway.
If you find serenity and happiness, they may be jealous;
Be happy anyway.
The good you do today, people will often forget tomorrow;
Do good anyway.
Give the world the best you have, and it may never be enough;
Give the world the best you've got anyway.
You see, in the final analysis, it is between you and your God;
It was never between you and them anyway

Half Locust Pose

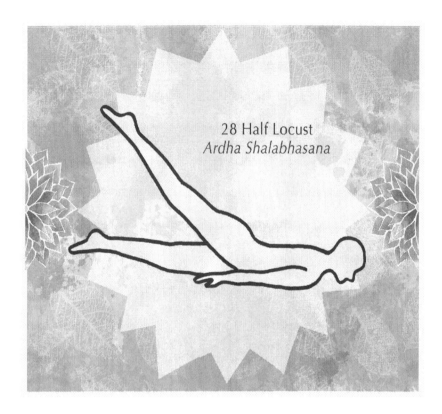

28 Half Locust
Ardha Shalabhasana

Builds strength along the spine, ignites the metabolism. Lift one leg as high as you can, do not strain the neck. Pause after each session.

The Yoga Teacher's Dog

Home from teaching yoga class
Body tingling, awake, feel the buzz
Feed my furry friends, walk them, talk to them,
hugs and kisses all around. Time to relax, cup of
de-tox tea
Crackers and a hunk of cheese.

Quietly as I check for messages and settle in
With laptop, table top, coffee pot, room hot,
beautiful spot in the sun. I look around for the
post-it note I used as a safe harbor for my hunk of
cheese....
Gone, gone, Sparky licking his chops waiting for
the next errant cheese morsel resting on a post-it
note.
Where was I when all this was going on?
Eyes glazed over, fixed on my computer screen
Missing the present moment. Darn!!!!
Gianna

Boat Pose

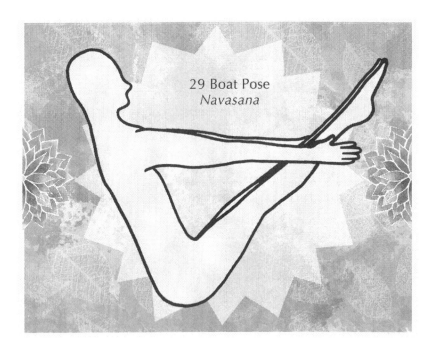

29 Boat Pose
Navasana

Fix your gaze, lift legs, engage the core, hold as long as you can. Release and go again.

Balance Is Key To Life

In everything you do keep balance.
Dance all night long and practice yoga the next
day.
Drink wine but don't forget your green juice.
Eat chocolate when your heart wants it and kale
salad when your body needs it.
Wear high heels on Saturday and walk barefoot on
Sunday.
Live high, live low, live loud, live quiet,
Move and stay still.
Embrace all sides of who you are.
Be brave, bold, spontaneous and reserved when
needed.
Dig deep to bring out your courage and go-for-the-
gold!
Aim for balance.
Make your own rules but do what is right.
Follow your path but every now and then take a
detour to what is unfamiliar.

Supine Twist

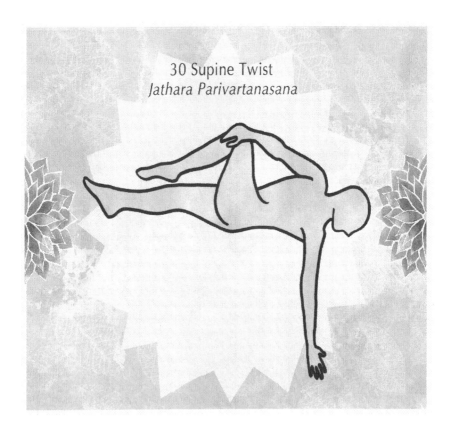

30 Supine Twist
Jathara Parivartanasana

Ahhh.. the divine release of the spine as you bend
one knee pull the knee across the body to the
opposite side, extend the other arm, turn your
gaze over the opposite shoulder.

Yoga Expands You

Your attention span is expanding.
Your imagination is stretching.
You are outgrowing your container.
Like a snake molting its skin.

It is time to trade in your claustrophobic cubicle
for a spacious new niche.
The boundaries you once knew
Are gone, you must transform.
We either grow or we wither,
atrophy and die.
The choice is that simple.

We make the choice every time we come
to the sacred space on our mats.
We make the choice to expand body
mind, breath and consciousness.

It is easy, listen to the teacher she will lead
you inward to encounter you again
but bigger, stronger and renewed.
Gianna

Supine Knee to Chest Pose

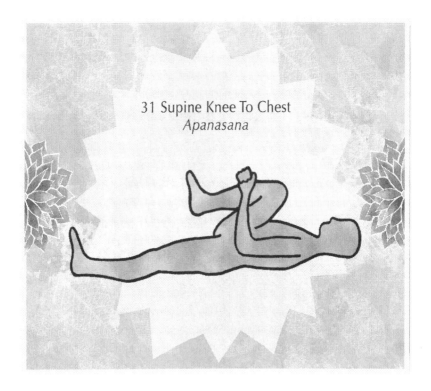

31 Supine Knee To Chest
Apanasana

Wind relieving pose but it also stretches the spine gently. Release the lumbar as you pull the shin closer to your body.

This Yoga Practice Heals Me

In tree pose, I am rooted, stand tall and allowed
my branches to grow toward the sun.
In sun salutations I honored the fire
And energy of the sun that creates, sustains and
nurtures.
In spinal twists I felt the inner wringing of clean,
serene abiding.
In mountain pose I witnessed my strength and
connection to the earth.
In Triangle I pushed out and over my hips, easing
to angle my body in perfect right angle alignment.
On the floor, I found divine release in a twist with
knees resting to each side. I found my spine
resting heavily on the bosom of mother earth. I felt
my spirit lift, connecting with all that is.
In Svasana I found "Ananda", pure bliss, as my
body rested and thanked me. My body resting
healing, absorbing new energy into my cells,
muscles and bones. The teacher invited us to
allow our bodies to absorb all the good work we
had done.
**Om…to the great universe, Om to those in my
tribe,….Om to my peaceful body. May we all
find peace, peace, peace!**

Side Plank Pose

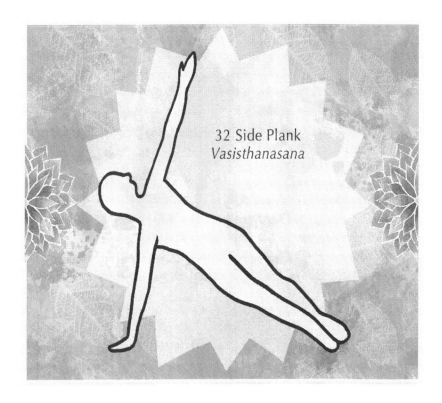

32 Side Plank
Vasisthanasana

From traditional plank roll to one side, stack your
feet if possible. Engage your core, don't slump.
Gaze skyward, breathe. You are stronger than you
think you are.

Another Lifetime, We'll Meet Again

You'll meet no strangers along the way, only the
old souls you knew earlier, in another lifetime.
You'll find grace in their words and wisdom in their
touch,
Nothing brings you home so much as this
recognition
Nothing compares to this unexplained encounter
of old friends from a lifetime ago
You say, I know this voice…it has spoken to me in
another language, in another land, a long time
ago.
And now, here, we are reunited as new/old friends
To face this time in the sand, moving grains with
our toes, how easy it is to know each other again.
"Welcome home my old friend" I say to myself.
"Welcome home."
Gianna for Margo

Tree Pose

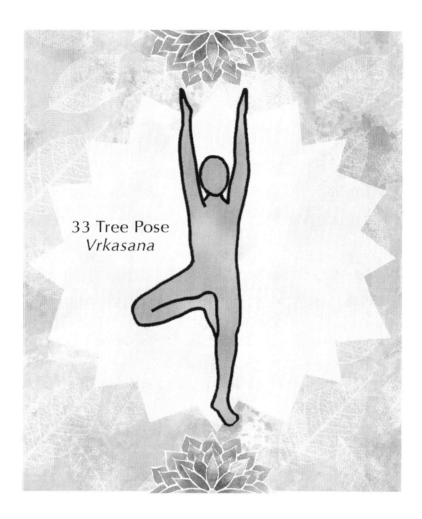

33 Tree Pose
Vrkasana

Root the standing leg strongly toward the earth,
pull the opposite foot either into the inner thigh or
at the ankle(never the knee), stare at your drishti,
then reach your arms as branches skyward.

Tree Pose

The tree is the ancient symbol of regeneration in many cultures.
It acts as a link stretching between the underworld, the earth and the heavens.
The roots coming up through the earth represent the unconscious or hidden aspects of the self-emerging into light. The trunk represents the strength of the spine and core.
The branches are consciousness reaching ever toward the light of enlightenment.
In yoga, Tree pose brings balance to the whole system.
Practicing Tree Pose, we feel the grounding of our feet, the strength of the trunk and the yielding nature of the leaves and branches as we reach our arms skyward towards the energy-giving light of the sun.
Then come the seasonal fluctuations of old leaves falling, a time of dormancy and then awakening with new leaves growing inspiring us to accept life's changes.
In Tree Pose, we honor the interconnection between human and plant life and experience the seeds of our own existence taking root and growing tall, branches ever reaching toward the light.

Goddess Pose

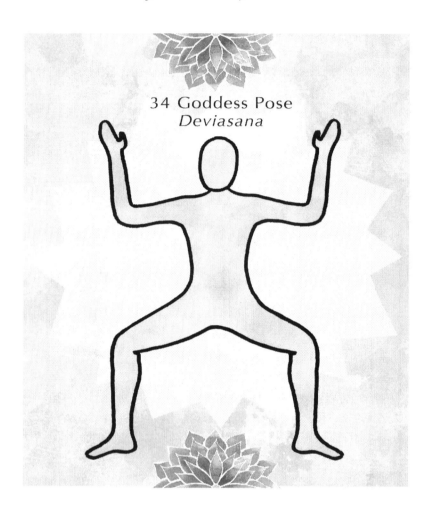

34 Goddess Pose
Deviasana

The legs are strong, muscles engaged from a wide stance bend the knees and drop you tailbone toward the earth. Arms are shoulder height bend elbows bringing hands skyward. Try to drop deeper into the pose.

Decision

When standing at the crossroads.
Presented with a choice
Listen within to the quiet voice,
It will help you find the path
That fulfills your dharma.

Easily, it unfolds, no drama, easy flow,
Lighting your way to go,
Each step is true to your nature, your purpose
unfolds.
You rest in this calm abiding,
Knowing the universe is on your side!
Om Shanti…Shanti….Shanti…

Bridge Pose

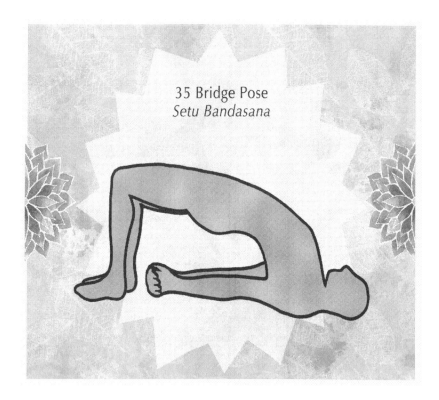

35 Bridge Pose
Setu Bandasana

Walk heels close to buttocks, interlace fingers behind your back and push knuckles toward the heels. Raise hips and chest skyward, breathe deeply. Hold for 10 breaths.

Think Like The Tiger

This story was told to me in Chennai, India, in a British hunting lodge at a tea plantation.

If you want to track a tiger, stay upwind.
Tie a goat to the stump of a tree.
Perceive the pattern of the thinking mind of the tiger.
Learn to notice the tracks and read the poop.
Learn where the wind blows, perceive the patterns of nature.
Don't get too close.
We pull back and perceive the entirety of the situation, the stump, the goat,
the tiger, the wind.
When we see the entire picture we can then be called to right action.
Gianna

Supine Knees to Chest Pose

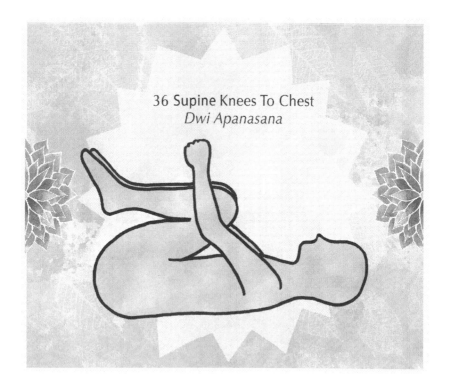

36 Supine Knees To Chest
Dwi Apanasana

Give yourself a big hug, rock side to side, close
your eyes.

Training Elephants In India

In India, they train baby elephants by tying one leg
to a sturdy tree.
At first it struggles and tries to escape. Eventually
it gives up, at that point the rope is untied and for
the rest of its life, that elephant never wanders
farther than the distance of the captive rope.
They never realize they are free!

The same for people;
in yoga, you come to a certain resistance, fatigue
or fear and your instincts say "This hurts…. I can't
do this… I have never done this before…I can't do
this…I am outta here."

But that my friends, is the moment of truth…that is
your chance for "break-through and growth!
For freedom from that psychological rope.
Say "yes" to transformation and growth!
This is when you view resistance as opportunities
for growth rather than a signal to quit.
Baron Baptiste

Seated Forward Fold

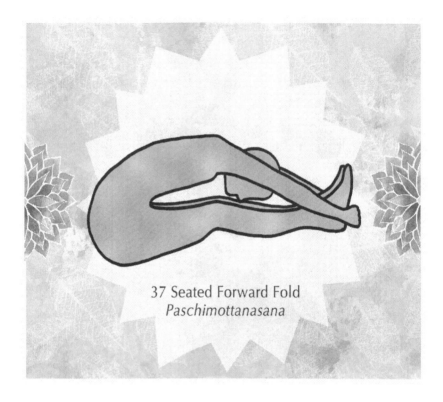

37 Seated Forward Fold
Paschimottanasana

As you elongate your legs, flex your feet, reach arms up, overhead, stretch then hinge at the hips and reach forward towards your feet. Elongate, breathes, be patient while the fascia and hamstrings release and relax.

In Yoga We Remember The Poses We Did As Children

We welcome the turn of the day by stretching upward then folding down into Sun Salutations, honoring the sun's energy, inviting it into our bodies to radiate, warm and heal.

What would life be like if we never took risks, never tried a headstand as we did as children. Remember the fun of rolling over on the front lawn as tried to stand on our heads in a balance?

What might we miss by backing away from the exploration of something we once did so freely as children?

We come to yoga not so much to "learn" but to "REMEMBER" what our bodies once did. Yoga reminds us of the body we once had and can now encounter once again every time we come to the mat.
Gianna

Seated Head to Knee Pose

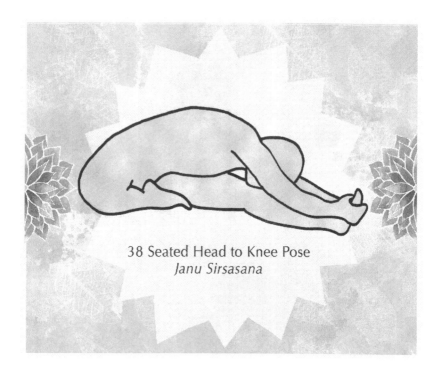

38 Seated Head to Knee Pose
Janu Sirsasana

One knee bent, foot into opposite thigh. Extend arms overhead to lengthen and then dive forward toward the extended leg. Reach chin toward toes, then surrender.

The Yoga Journey Inward

The journey inward is a personal one and not always easy. We discover places in our bodies that were so root-bound or rock hard that we have to chip away at them gingerly because we are afraid of breaking. In the beginning, we are unsure of the poses, we fear hurting our spine, or our neck, but then we discover how strong we really are or in some cases, how weak. When first doing shoulder stand or plow we feel strained. In Fish, we feel the strange stretch of our neck... We are lucky when we have a compassionate and experienced teacher who teaches with a sense of play and joy. We learn how to let go of fears and even how to do a balance pose or a headstand. In the process we release acres of emotional residue that years of therapy and various forms of healing had chipped away at but not yet unearthed. We may have done aerobics, running or martial arts, yet we find Yoga is the one practice that allowed us a deep, meditative experience into the body and mind. Breath by breath we allow ourselves to unfold into yoga again and again. We explore ourselves petal by petal like the lotus flower that quietly opens to the sunlight. Then one day if our practice is sincere, we are there, at home, gazing into the beautiful heart of the lotus we call our body.

Rolf Gates, Meditations from The Mat

Bow Pose

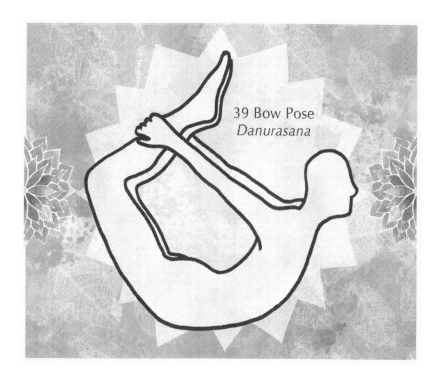

39 Bow Pose
Danurasana

Lying prone bend one leg at a time reaching back grabbing the ankle or foot. Rest for a moment take an inhale and on the exhale, push your legs into your hands gently arching the back, lifting chest-chin, roll shoulders back, gaze forward. Breathe 5 – 10 breaths. Lower down, release feet, notice the beating of your heart. Give thanks.

Understanding Yourself

The magic of going inward is that it can take us
away from our busy selves.
The breath becomes the bridge to greater self-
understanding, to calming the mind, which leads to
deeper understanding of not only ourselves but of
others.
The postures in yoga are simply a means to get
us out of the thinking mind and into the "resting"
mind and thus fully integrate into the heart and
spirit.

In yoga we encounter our resistance and our
ability to forge ahead.
We shake hands with challenge, we make friends
with fears, and we let go of anxiety.
Every step, in self-acceptance loosens reins of
doubt.
We find we are much stronger than we think we
are.
We are more flexible in mind and body than we
remembered.
With time and practice we understand the
evolution and surrender into it.
We give thanks for the body we live in.

ℱish 𝒫ose

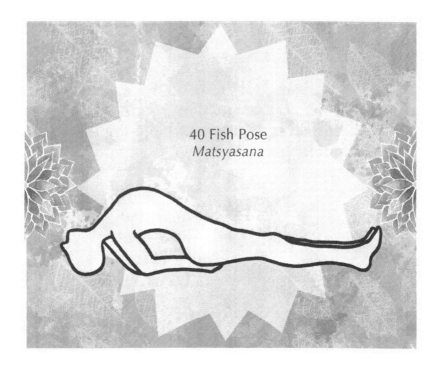

40 Fish Pose
Matsyasana

Resting in supine, place hands under buttocks, lift to your elbows, allow your head to roll back so that the crown of the head rests on the floor. Your gaze is behind you, let your lips part if necessary. Breathe deeply feeling the expansion of the chest with each of the 5 – 10 breaths.

Embracing The Process And Not The Goal

We find that our yoga practice gives is patience
and takes us away from the focus on the "goal".
It gets us into a deeper appreciation of the
"process", away from the "doing" and into "being".

Yoga moves us away from thinking and into "pure
experience", into trust and sometimes into
complete joy.

The record keeper of the universe knows the value
of listening. We listen to our bodies and then let
our bodies abide in the pose, our breath taking us
deeper.
Then we notice what comes up in the stillness.
What do we embrace?
What can we let go of?

This is our personal journey on the mat toward
acceptance, patience, forgiveness and grace.

Each pose gives us a new opportunity to explore
and receive a gift from us, to ourselves.
Namaste

Pigeon Pose

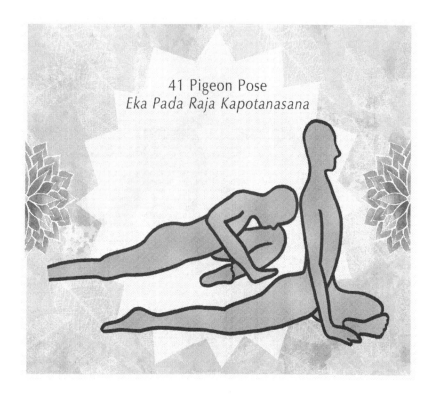

41 Pigeon Pose
Eka Pada Raja Kapotanasana

Pigeon Pose, the ultimate pose for dealing with inner demons that reside in our hips. We harbor all the disappointments, trauma and unresolved events in our hips. This is the opportunity to let them go and free up the tension. From Down Dog, sweep the knee forward, bring it behind the wrist or between your hands whichever is available to you. Lift your torso, big inhale, then lower upper torso over the extended knee. Let all the weight of your body melt over the extended thigh. Breathe.. It is okay to cry.

The Paradox Of Our Times….

….Is that we have taller buildings, but shorter
tempers.
Wider freeways, but narrower viewpoints.
We spend more, but we have less.
We have bigger houses, but smaller families.
More conveniences, but less time.
We have more degrees, but less sense.
More knowledge, but less judgement.
More experts, but more problems.
More medicines, but less wellness.
We have multiplied our possessions, but reduced
our values.
We talk too much, love too seldom, and hate too
often.
We have learnt how to make a living, but not a life.
We have added years to life, but not life to years.
We've been all the way to the moon and back
But have trouble crossing the street to meet the
new neighbor.
We have conquered outer space, but not inner
space.

We've cleaned up the air, but polluted our soul.
We've split the atom, but not our prejudice.
We've higher incomes, but lower morals.
We've become long on quantity but short on quality.
These are the times of tall men, and short character;
Steep profits, and shallow relationships.
These are the times of world peace, but domestic warfare,
More leisure, but less fun; more kinds of food, but less nutrition.
These are the days of two incomes, but more divorces;
Of fancier houses, but broken homes.
It is a time when there is much in the show window, and nothing in the stockroom.

- His Holiness, The Dalai Lama -

The Supreme Guru lives within.

Never miss an opportunity to sing...
Singing cleanses the soul.

May all beings be free of suffering.
Never kill the happiness of a living being.
Buddha

The right side of the heart is where God
waits for you.
Light of the Atman

Relax with what is....
Adversity reveals your genius.
Horace

Supine Hand to Toe Pose

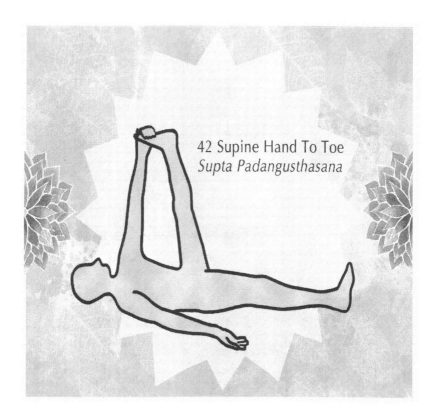

42 Supine Hand To Toe
Supta Padangusthasana

Lying down, extend one leg out on the floor raise the other leg, try to keep the leg straight. Grab the big toe with your first two fingers, push away with the heels, gently pull the airborne leg down to the floor beside you, Airplane opposite arm, rest, breathe feel the inner thigh release.

NATURE TEACHES US

Yoga encourages us to be outside with nature as often as possible. And when you are, rather than sit on a bench, sit on the ground or a rock so that your body connects with the elements of earth.
Then....
Be like the Sun – Be your own illumination!
Be like the Birds – Sing your heart out!
Be like the Stream – Do not stop for any obstacles but flow over and around them.
Be like the trees – When the wind blows bend easily and trust your roots to hold.
Be like the Galaxy – Remember your vastness.
Be like the Ant – Small does not mean powerless.
Be like the Clouds – Float gently knowing the sun is there behind you.
Be Silent – In the quiet all becomes clear and the answers appear.

Low Lunge Twist

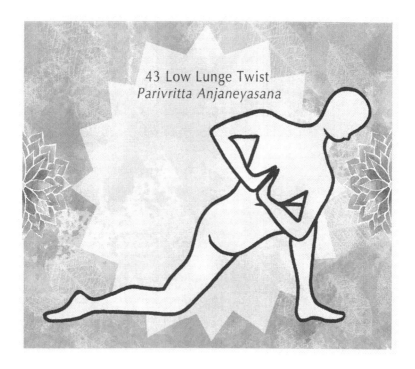

43 Low Lunge Twist
Parivritta Anjaneyasana

From Forward Fold, send one leg as far back on your mat as possible, coming down onto the back knee and a back foot. Reach arms skyward, bring hands to prayer and twist over the forward thigh. Feel the squeeze through your mid-section, cleansing the inner organs.

Let The Body Move With Spirit And Breath

As we deepen our yoga practice we are asked to
get out of our own way and let the body move with
spirit and breath.
As the body and heart open so do the channels of
creativity and grace.
We find that the exploration of any given pose is
as important-if-not more-so than the execution of a
picture-perfect-posture.
It can be wonderful to fall, roll over, to pick oneself
up and try again.
It is then we learn about our own capacity for
resiliency both on the mat and in life.

Yogic Squat

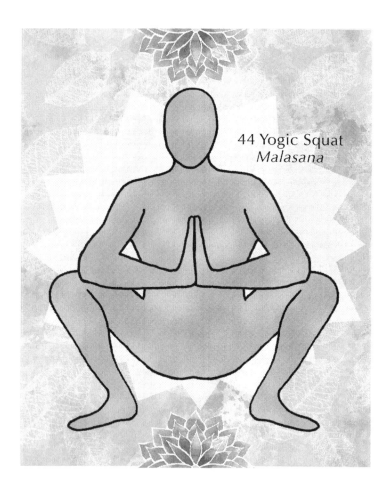

44 Yogic Squat
Malasana

From a wide stance, bring the tailbone toward the floor as deeply as you can while still off the floor. Bring hands together at Anjali Mudra, dig elbows into inside of knees to intensify the inner thigh stretch. Straighten your spine, close eyes, breathe.

Align Your Life With The "Spirit"

When you consciously align your life with "spiritual
law," you are asking the universe to support and
guide you with success and abundance.

The earlier someone cultivates the "spirit" the
earlier life becomes effortless, harmonious,
creative.
Then it is more likely that all of life will bring
effortless success.
With spirit we are all children of the cosmos,
without it we are orphaned and set adrift.

We need to be strong enough of spirit to withstand
the harsh realities of an often, un-spiritual world.

Taking a moment to breathe before reacting with
give the spirit a chance to come to the forefront of
every action; that is when the spirit speaks and
guides the response.

Crow Pose Balance

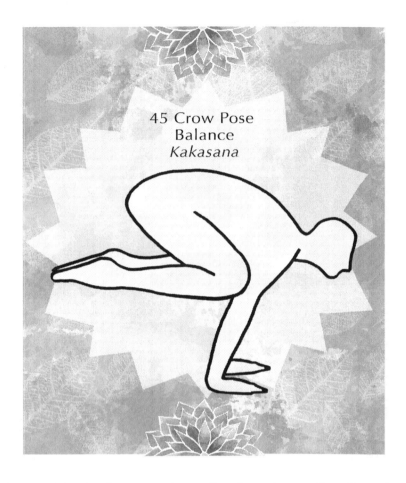

45 Crow Pose
Balance
Kakasana

From Yogic Squat, place the hands on the floor in front of your feet hip distance apart. Spread your fingers. Ride your knees up the back of your arms above the elbows, lift your face and begin to look forward as you lean forward placing more and more weight onto your upper arms. Smile as your feet take flight.

Autumn

Autumn offers us an invitation to balance the polarities between tension and relaxation.

When leaves turn, fields and gardens are harvested and temperatures begin to drop we are reminded on a daily basis that *nothing is permanent*, everything is fleeting.

For some, we lean into the seasonal wave and passionately thrive off change.
The unknown brings us inspiration, as around the next corner is potent opportunity waiting to be explored.
For others, we resist the seasonal shift and cling to summer like the last leaf on a bare tree.
Change creates friction.
It is a reminder of things lost, moments ended and time that we can never get back.
But lest we forget,
that change in weather brings new opportunities, the quietness of the season brings us indoors, closer to friends and loved ones.
Warm meals and chilly nights.
We have renewed appreciation for the energy and warmth of the sun as we hold vigil for the winter.

Camel Pose

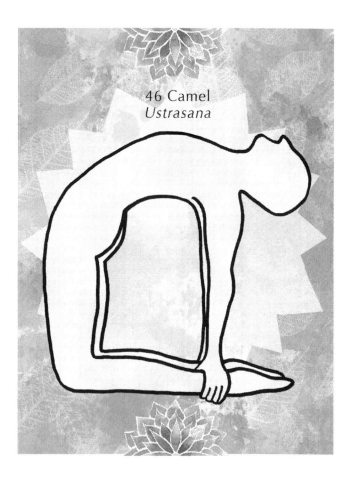

46 Camel
Ustrasana

On your knees if you have trouble reaching back to your ankles curl your toes under and rest your hands on your heels as you lean back and gaze skyward.

Camel Pose

Like the desert animal, we can replenish when
resources are low or we feel depleted.
Camel pose celebrates the opening of the heart.
Back bending is often bumpy terrain and requires
faith.
This graceful pose transforms our habitual
tendency to hunch forward looking over our
cellphones and computers.
Camel Pose helps us to reach our full potential for
joy and opening to grace.
Camel Pose cultivates patience with ourselves
and joy by opening the heart toward the sky.
Through this practice we tap into the large reserve
of energy within ourselves. We discover our own
ability to self-nourish and replenish.

Shoulder Stand

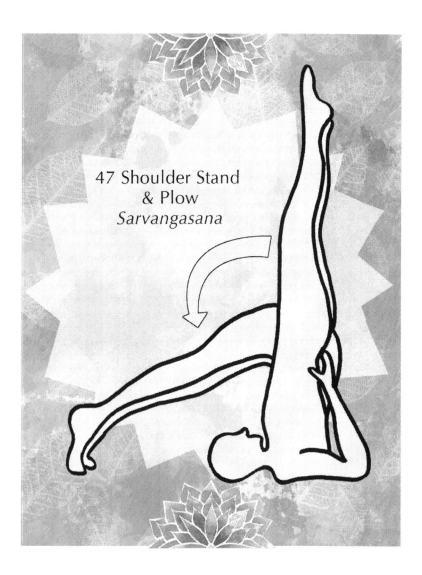

47 Shoulder Stand
& Plow
Sarvangasana

Raise legs, rest on shoulders (a folded blanket under shoulders helps). Squeezes thyroid, moves the biochemistry around, helps lymphatic system.

98

Abundance

The source of all abundance is not outside you...It is part of who you are.
Start by acknowledging and recognizing the abundance within and without.
See the fullness of life all around. The warmth of the sun on your skin.
The display of magnificent flowers outside, biting into a succulent fruit, or getting soaked in the rain, honor the abundance of water falling from the sky as a gift of life.
The fullness of life is there at every step.
The acknowledgement of that abundance that is all around you awakens the dormant abundance within. Then let it flow out.
When you smile at a stranger, there is already a generous outflow if energy.
You become a giver, ask yourself often "What can I give here, how can I be of service to this person or this situation?"
You don't need to own anything to feel abundant, although, if you feel abundant consistently things will almost certainly come to you.
Abundance comes only to those who already have it. It sounds unfair but it is a universal law.
Both abundance and scarcity are inner states that manifest as your reality.
Chose abundance every time.

Reverse Plank Pose

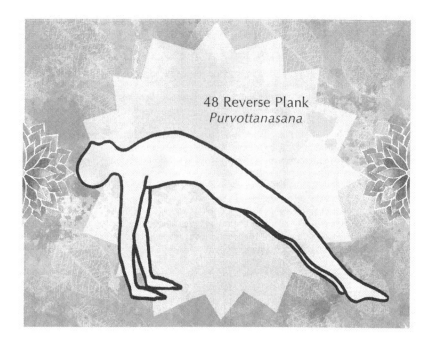

48 Reverse Plank
Purvottanasana

Opens the thoracic region, builds strength in the upper body and core, strengthens the calves and thighs. Breath, gaze skyward, let your head fall back.

Leaving Last Year And Sliding Into The New Year

Time to say good bye to what was, now we greet what will be.
For now, the present is all we have, we exist in this space between the past and the future.
No regrets, just lessons learned. No sorrows to weigh us down but songs and sunlight to keep us young.
Looking back only strains the neck. Predicting forward only strains the heart.
Living now with wholeness of attention will make us new.
Let us create random acts of kindness.
Let us fling the past into the trunk. Let us learn to give more and take less.
Let us cherish what we have and leave alone what does not serve.
Let us spend more time with loved ones and good friends. Less time with those who do not cherish what is.
Let us see the blessings in all that we receive.
Let us send blessings in all that we give.
Let us see the sacred in the sunlight, in a child's eyes, works of art
and the moon at night.
Be inspired to write more, love more, give more.

Stay careful to tread lightly on our sacred planet.
Pollute not.
Be proud to bend and pick up some fluttering
debris.
Keep Clean your mind and body.
Keep your heart full by shining light into dark
spaces.
Be uplifting, less critical, be supportive, be kind,
less cold, be aware and awake, be less asleep, be
grateful, less entitled.
Let all things occur in their own time, don't rush
into life, take the time to savor.
Be grateful, and say so often.
The New Year is here let us celebrate!!!

In meditation we become action-less, we lose the sensation of the body so that the soul may be revealed.
Tibetan saying

The breath leads one to meditation. Meditation leads one to the soul.

Self-realization comes with purity of heart.
Dharma Mittra

Compassion is the first step towards enlightenment.
Eating animals shows lack of compassion.

The cow lives her life shedding milk and tears.

Double Pigeon

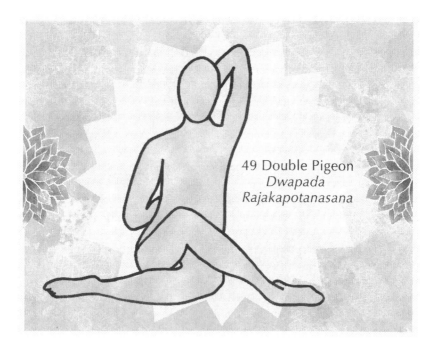

49 Double Pigeon
*Dwapada
Rajakapotanasana*

Sometimes called Cow Face Pose, the top arm reaches down the back to clasp the hand of the lower arm opening the shoulder joint. The top leg crosses over the bottom knee to open hip joints. Breathe, find calm abiding.

Find The Hidden Harmony In Chaos

When we go into a forest that has not been
interfered with by man, our thinking mind will see
only disorder and chaos all around us.
We won't even be able to differentiate between life
and death anymore since everywhere new life
grows out of rotting and decaying matter.

Only if we are still enough inside and the
noise of thinking subsides can we become aware
that there is a hidden harmony here,
a sacredness, a higher order in which
everything has its perfect place and balance
and could not be other than what it is and
the way it is.

Supine Bound Angle Pose

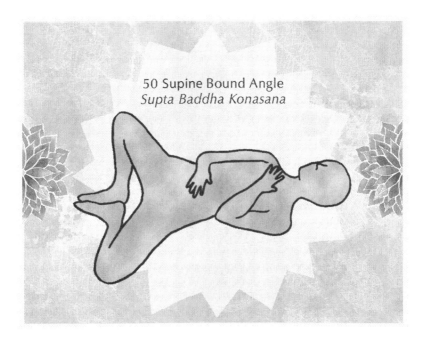

50 Supine Bound Angle
Supta Baddha Konasana

We know the class will be ending soon. This pose allows our joints to surrender into gravity. Soles of feet are touching, knees splayed apart, hands resting on heart and belly chakra. Our breath is long and sweet, we surrender, relax, let the body be as though a frog who is resting in the sunlight, belly up.
Have faith in the body to heal.

Reaching The Cosmic Ocean Of Energy

The 3rd eye is awakened as we flood the nerve
channels with the pranic energy of deep breathing.

This pranic energy sends a shower of light through
every cell of our being.

In this moment the union of Shiva and Shakti
merge,
There is an explosion of joy,
A convergence of beauty, bounty and blessings
This is the union of sun and moon, yin and yang
male and female, fire and water.

The walls of duality crumble and
all becomes one!
The empty mind merges into oneness,
bathing in divine bliss.
This becomes the culmination of the true sense of
Yoga, union, yoking together!

Where the rivers of breath-energy from all
parts of our being culminate
and flow into the Cosmic Ocean of Energy.

We become one with all that Is.
We rest knowing that we are part of
the great Cosmic Plan.

Final Relaxation Pose

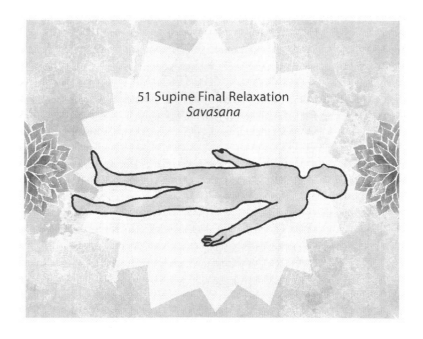

51 Supine Final Relaxation
Savasana

Resting in supine takes great courage, we surrender doing into being as we come to Sssssssavasana...

This is the most IMPORTANT pose of our practice, where we allow the body to absorb and metabolize, all the good work we have done. We totally melt into the cracks of the floor, we allow every bone and muscle to relax, our breathing becomes normal. This is the sweet surrender of peaceful conclusion.

In This Darkened Room
- Modified

In this darkened room, thoughts have slipped through
me,
Through the cracks in the floor, through vertebrae
tingling,
Joints loose, hips liberated.
I lay under the yoga blanket, eyes closed, lavender
floating in the air makes its way through my nostrils.
Deep breath ceased, shallow breathing now.
I have forgotten my errands for the week.
I am aware of a car sloshing through the puddles
outside.
I am interrupted by a person's untimely cough.
I am pondering my regrets.
I am melancholy remembering my departed friend.
I am planning which tea to drink after my practice.
Still..... I lay perfectly still. I am perfectly
warm and cool,
I have found equilibrium in this moment.
"Find your Dristhi" the teacher says,
yes, I have found it.
I lay feeling my lower back and measure its
ache and release.
My pelvis is grateful for the attention.
I have learned to love my body.
My feet are relieved to be done with their job of
holding me up, rooting me into
Warrior poses and forward folds.
Shoulders and neck aching from
the **dogs** carried upward and downward.

From **Mountains** erected, muscles engaged.
Balancing Trees stretched toward the sky.
Greeting and **salutations** to the sun!
Legs proving their strength by holding me up steady
to stand in **warrior** and **triangle,**
Then to sit with **pigeons**, hip joints opening,
old fears flying away.
Breathing, melting through the pose.
Next time I will go deeper, I will stay just a little longer
in the pose.
And just as I am letting my thoughts flow
through the creases of my mind
Guru rings a gentle bell.
Three times it resonates louder.
It tugs me back into reality.
I stretch, reach, and roll over letting all that concerns
me fall to the side. I am happy, Ananda bliss has
come.
I rise. My body levitates upwards. My eyes are still
closed, in dark awareness.
I feel and sense others around me, I hear their
stirrings.
We chant Om, 3 times, it vibrates in my throat and
heart Om ...seals our practice and our prayers.
Namaste to the light of the teacher and to light
within...**Namaste to the light of all.**
And all those things I thought I needed to do,
The worries and distractions, are left in the cracks of
the floor.
I leave the yoga womb refreshed and renewed. My
mind is calm but my body is alert. I am home.

Fear prevents one from fully softening into
the possible.

A state of profound loving requires
a softening of the heart and soul.

Namaste Meaning
"The light in me honors the light in you."

Seated Lotus Pose

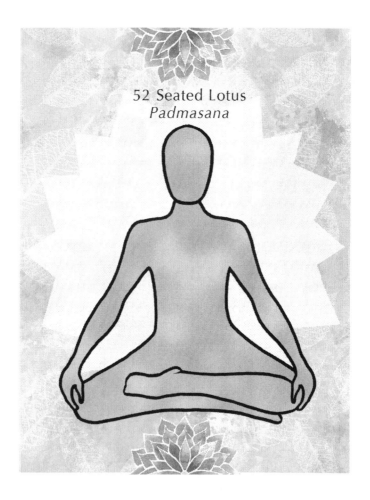

52 Seated Lotus
Padmasana

The ritual of Lotus pose brings us up to seated, we rest with eyes closed, we bring hands together at prayer to ask for peace, blessings and grace. We quietly remember the ones we love and those we've yet to love.
Namaste, Om Shanti

Savasana

I lay in Peace
The only peace I have known all day,
The one peaceful moment I own.
I feel myself falling through the cracks in the floor.
My yoga mat has become one with my body.
My jaw relaxes into deep release I begin to float.
The Tibetan bowls ring
Once, twice...third time.
The sound is distant.
I am semi-conscious.
I try to will away the sound of bowls,
I try to will away the scuffling in the room.
Someone coughs.
In a distance I hear guru say: "Come to seated and
bring your hands together in prayer".
Am I dreaming? I am lost in my stillness,
In the only perfect stillness I own.
In the distance I hear stirring,
I am riding soft clouds of dreamless sleep
Am I being called back?
I am invited to sit up, cross- legged.
I resist, but then I re-enter consciousness,
Re-enter my body.
Follow the invitation to sit up, to chant Om
To collect my things and move out into the
Dark cold night.
Startled awake, but deep inside rested.
Tomorrow there will be stillness again.
Danna Faulds

Oṃ

Oṃ

Om is a Sanskrit Chant used at the beginning and end of yoga practice. It is written in Sanskrit like a number three with a curved tail to it symbolizing the sub-conscious world and the crescent shape above with dot symbolizing the divine consciousness.

Om is the audible expression of the transcendental call to the universe. *Om* is the "primordial seed" of the universe. It is believed that the whole world, is made of the vibrating sound of *Om*. It is the root mantra from which all other mantras emerge.

In Christianity the sound is **Amen**. If you drone the sound of **Aaaa**.....and then end with **...men** it becoming a relative of *Om*. In the Hebraic texts there is **Shalom** encompassing the seed sound **Om** once again. The closing "mmm..." sound creates a vibration in the heart chakra which reflects the center from which the Divine emanates. In Arabic there is **Salaam**, once again droning the ending double "a" and "m" sound. When sounding OM a vibration is created in the thoracic region which reveals the will of the heart, as the sound leaves the body it connects to the cosmic energy of all creation.

Chanting Om

Chanting Om is a collective act, a method of centering and connecting with others from the heart. Hands at prayer (Anjali Mudra) bring heart awareness into the center of your body while you are in the company of others in this room. Know that as your heart beats, so their hearts beat. Listen to the harmony of the voices around you, Om is not a selfish act but an act of harmony with others. Take a deep inhale and let the exhale be OMmmm....
Then bow your head in service to your heart.

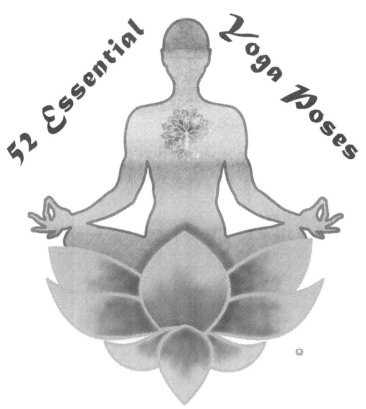

The Significance Of The Lotus Flower

Sitting on the lotus flower is an enlightened being.

The Lotus flower is the national flower of India and its radiant beauty represents spiritual growth. Contemplate the path of the lotus flower, whose life begins at the bottom of muddy, dark swamp rivers and ponds. Its stem extends from the swamp bottom sometimes as long as 22 feet, drawing nourishment from the murky depths, pushing its flower bud ever upward toward the light. Once at the surface of the water the morning sun opens its radiant petals until about 3p.m. During that time the channels and waterways of are a carpet of delicate, pastel waxy flowers. Once they close in the afternoon, the rivers go green again with a carpet of leaf ponds floating atop the water.

For Indians and Yogis who meditate, the lotus flower represents enlightenment. Reaching a state of Samadhi (inner peace), deep meditative contemplation, opening the mind is related to the opening of the lotus flower. All depictions of Buddha and "enlightened beings" are of them sitting atop of open lotus flower.

The lotus flower ever reaching toward the "light" (enlightenment) from the murky bottoms, remains radiantly pristine, in the same manner that you can bring the beauty of your soul to shine in the chaos of your daily life, and that you can rise above the murkiness of life and find your own light.

ABOUT THE AUTHOR

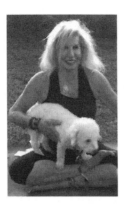

Joan (Gianna) Ragona-Suarez
*500hour E-RYT Experienced-Registered Yoga
Instructor and Yoga Teacher Trainer.*

Gianna is trained in the classic Hatha Vinyasa Style of Yoga and is deeply committed to bringing the practice of yoga in its purest and best form to those who seek transformation and evolution.

In 2012, she quit her corporate job in finance and purchased *Go Yoga Amelia Island Yoga Studio* where she taught and provided Yoga Teacher Training. She has volunteered for Wounded Warriors and worked with cancer patients, and the Boys and Girls Clubs.

Over the past twenty-four years, Gianna has trained in various styles including Lotus Gardens, Dharma Mittra, Lokenath, Sivananda in Uruguay, Yoga Den, Retreats in Tuscany, Omega Institute and Kripalu.

After 6 years of "island life", Gianna sold *Go Yoga Amelia Island* and moved to The Villages, Fl, where she continues to teach and write.

You may write to her at:*Yogaconcepts@gmail.com*

**Footnote from Gianna's daughter:

"We have a responsibility to our home, this planet, as yogis, to lead the way to a greater, deeper connection with our living, breathing Earth. I believe that is important to live in a way that sustains the planet for future generations. If yogis are not part of the global change then who will be?"
Celine M. Suarez

Great gratitude to Janet Michea who enhanced my artwork and made it beautiful. To Nancy Hellekson, yogi, literary expediter and computer genie, who brought it all together for this book. To all the students over the years who showed up on their mats and took the journey with me, who inspired me and had faith in the amazing, healing process of this ancient discipline we call yoga. To all of you, Namaste, I have seen and honor your light.

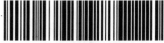

26594267R00077

Made in the USA
Lexington, KY
31 December 2018